Fighting To Move

Parkinson's disease

This is my story❤ ☐ This is my song

This book tells of the many painful, debilitating symptoms that come with (Pd), and the very harmful side effects of the medicine given to those with Parkinson's disease

Diagnosis

My family doctor noticed that I had no swing in my right arm. I also had a limp in my right leg

I had gone to the doctor because I was having tremors in my right hand. My doctor made me an appointment with a neurologist

The neurologist confirmed the diagnosis was Parkinson's disease

My Enemy is time

At around the seventh year I started getting different kinds of symptoms. I found it harder to walk. It was getting where it was hard to move my hands. My fingers felt like rubber bands .I knew my (pd) was getting worse . I started experiencing a lot of falls. It seemed my feet would just fall out from beneath me.

I would drop things for no reason It seemed that once the symptoms started. They came on closer together When I started to lose my ability to walk. I wanted to give up. I hated the sight of my wheel chair. I could walk a few steps but my legs just wouldn't go. My legs felt like they weighed 20 lbs each. I didn't want to go to church any more or to any place people were gathered. I was ashamed of my tremors. I was even more ashamed of my stiff face and body

I became very angry at God,I thought to myself. How can a loving and merciful God allow so much pain.. I tried to live for you . Now look at me. Where are you God I would pray. It seemed that God had forsaken me. My Grandfather was a Baptist minister.Grandfather was the reason I knew about healing and all the other miracles Jesus performed while on earth. When I was 15 my mom changed her denomination to the Assembly of God. The Assembly of God Church was known for their belief in healing and miracles. They preach the true living word of God.

After being angry at God for two years, and let go of my self pity. I started thinking about God. How good he has been to me. And the many times he healed my kids, myself and my husband. I finally repented of my anger and self pity. I invited Jesus back in my life. Not that he had left me. I turned from him. But he welcomed me back with open arms. This is my story. This is my song, praising my savior all the day long.

Husband Healed

My husband and I had not been married long when he had his first kidney stone. Some X-rays were taken of his kidneys . The X-ray showed a mass in one of his kidney's. We were very concerned about this mass. My brother and I put our hand on him and prayed for his healing, The next morning they did more X-rays . The doctor came in to talk to my husband. He said. Mr. Anglin. I don't know what happened on your X-rays from yesterday. That mass I was telling you about , Well it is gone. Today we took more X-rays. there is no mass. God still heals

There are two kinds of healings
1.When God performs a instant healing that's a miracle   2. there is a gradual healing where the person is healed but not miraculously. This is a gradual healing. It may take weeks are months before the healing is complete. They gradually get better over time.

I don't know the reason God works like he doe's . Everything that happens there is a purpose .

Who are we to tell God anything. God is the potter. We are the clay. He molds us and makes us what he wants us to be.

Two years ago I was healed

I was home alone listening to praise and worship music. I felt like Jesus was

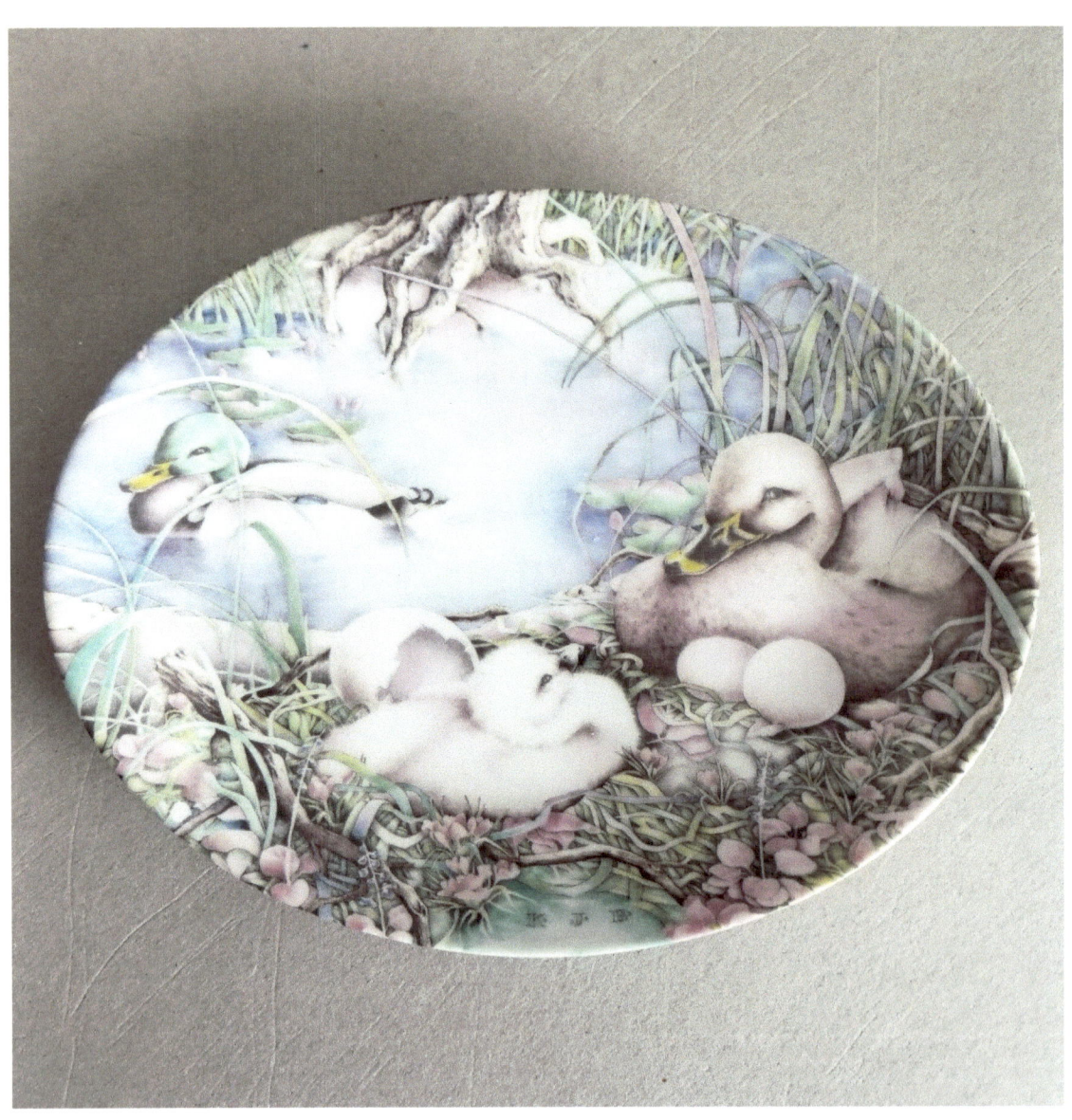

telling me to get up. I stood up from my chair. The Spirit of God filled the room . Gods spirit was so strong, like a stormy wind .I could hear the spirit of God whisper in my heart so gentle , but yet with authority.You are healed from this disease

I didn't feel like I was healed. It wasn't a bolt of lightening and thunder. Just a sweet aroma.Like when Jesus walks into a room. When I first wake up in the mornings my tremors are the worst. It takes about an hour for the tremors to go away.

This morning everything was different .No tremors. I waited for the tremors to return. They never did come back with the same intensity as before.

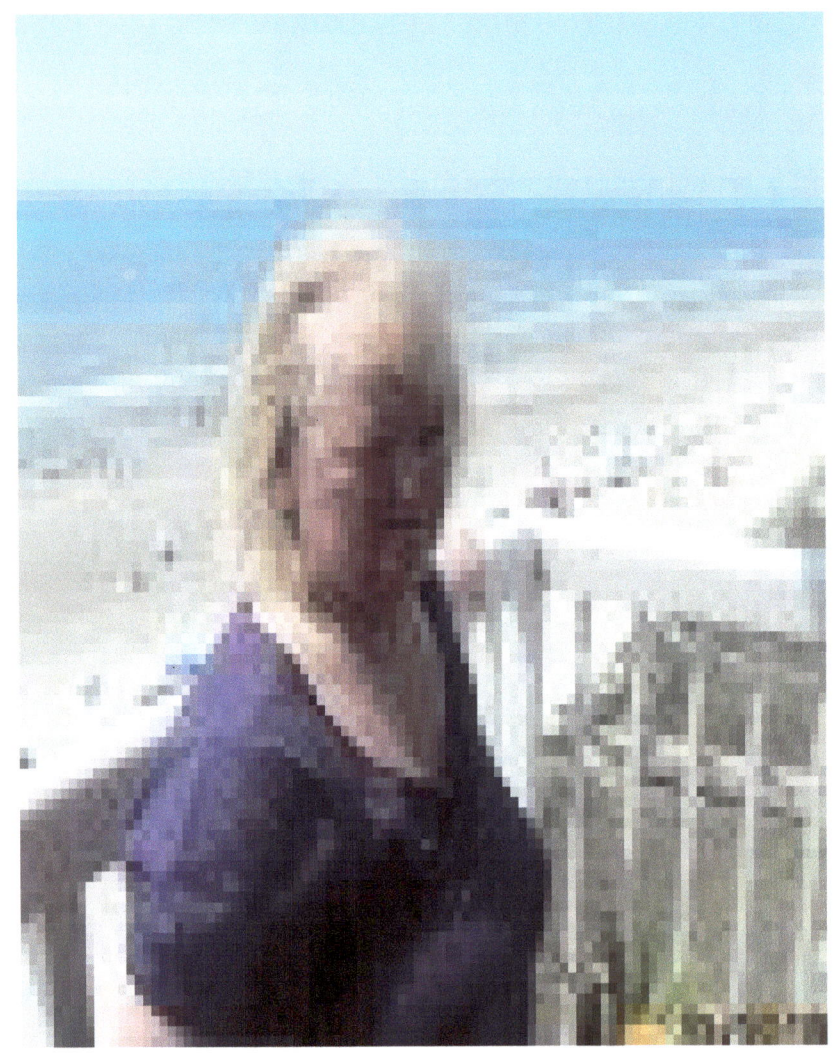

I am about 80 per cent better now

. People with Parkinson's disease lose hope because there is no cure for this chronic condition

I am here to tell you that there is hope. I'm not telling you that God will heal you. I can tell you that if I had not known Jesus as my savior I would not have made it.

When I felt the lowest and I didn't think I could go on another day, Jesus always brought me out and renewed my mind

Trust him. He said he would never leave nor forsake us. Jesus said that he would be with us always even to the end.

Things you can't change or do anything about. Give them to Jesus. He said he would carry our burdens for us.

Faith

With out faith it is impossible to please God

Taste and see that God is good

Arise and be healed

I am the God who heals you of all your diseases

I will bless your going and your coming.

Arise and be healed

I can do all things through Christ who strengthens me

Jesus Christ the same today, yesterday and forever

Trust in the lord with all your heart and he will guide your foot steps

Let not your heart be troubled

The peace of God that passes all understanding shall keep our hearts and minds through Christ Jesus our Lord

God will keep us in perfect peace whose mind is stayed on him.

Me and my husband

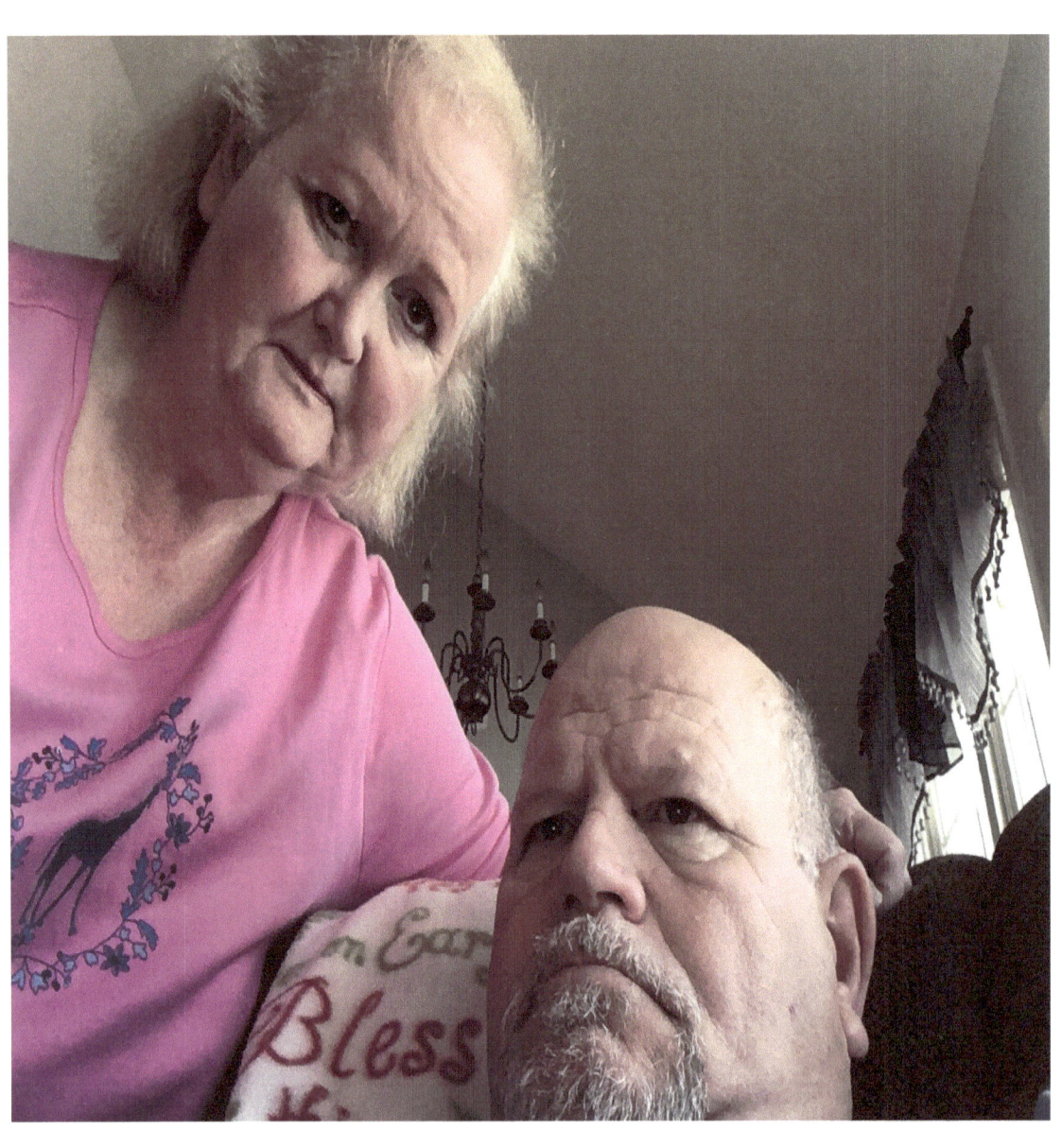

I dedicate this book to my husband : Sidney Anglin

My three kids Teresa, Amanda and Shane

My two grand children. Emily and Bryson

I thank all of you for taking care of me and being there for me

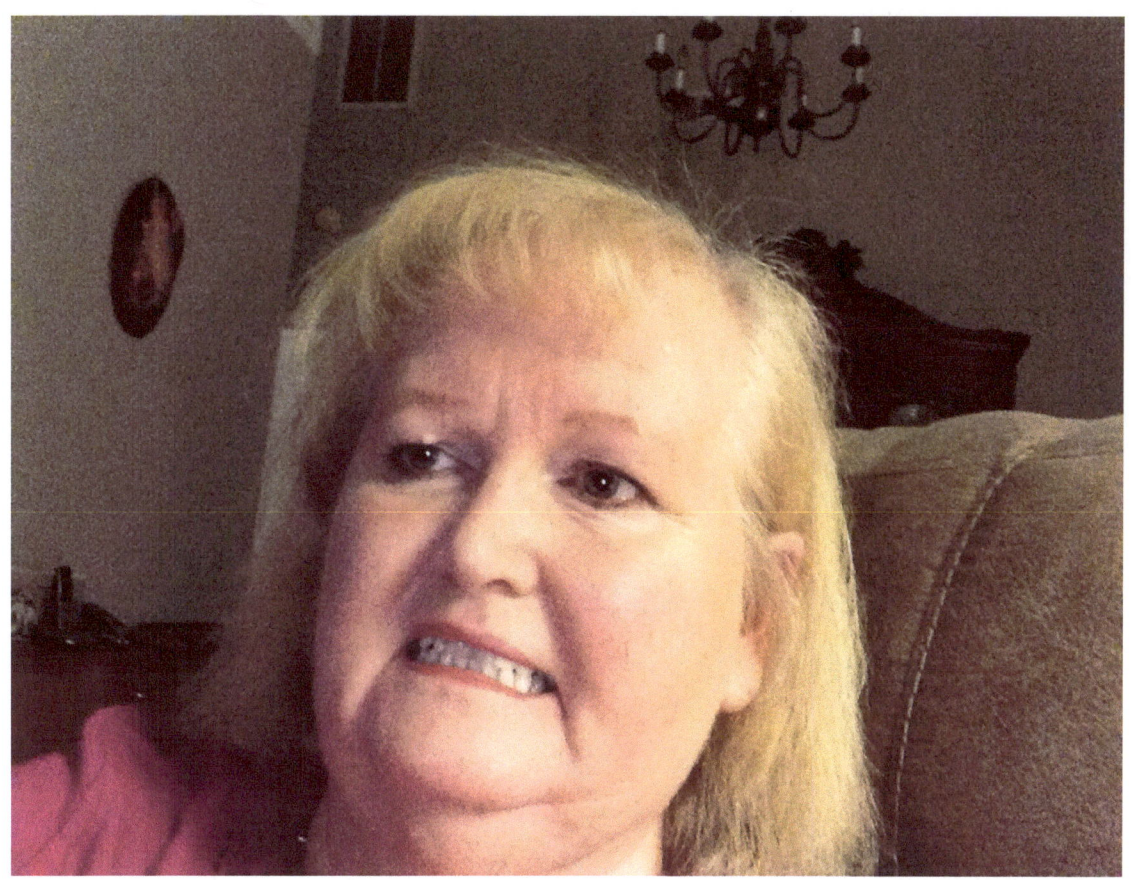
Me

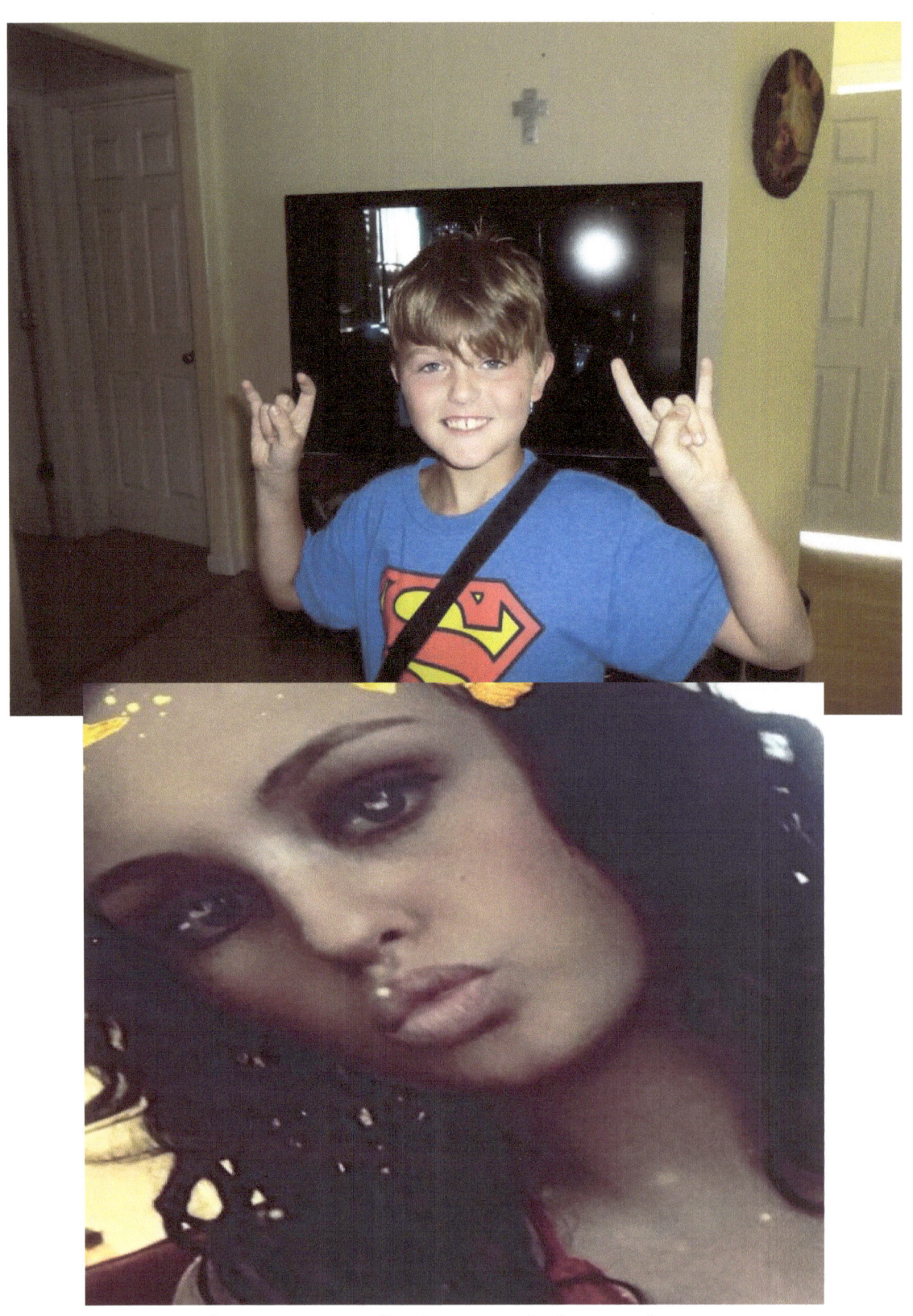

My grandson and Granddaughter

This is the day that the Lord has made.
I will rejoice and be glad in it

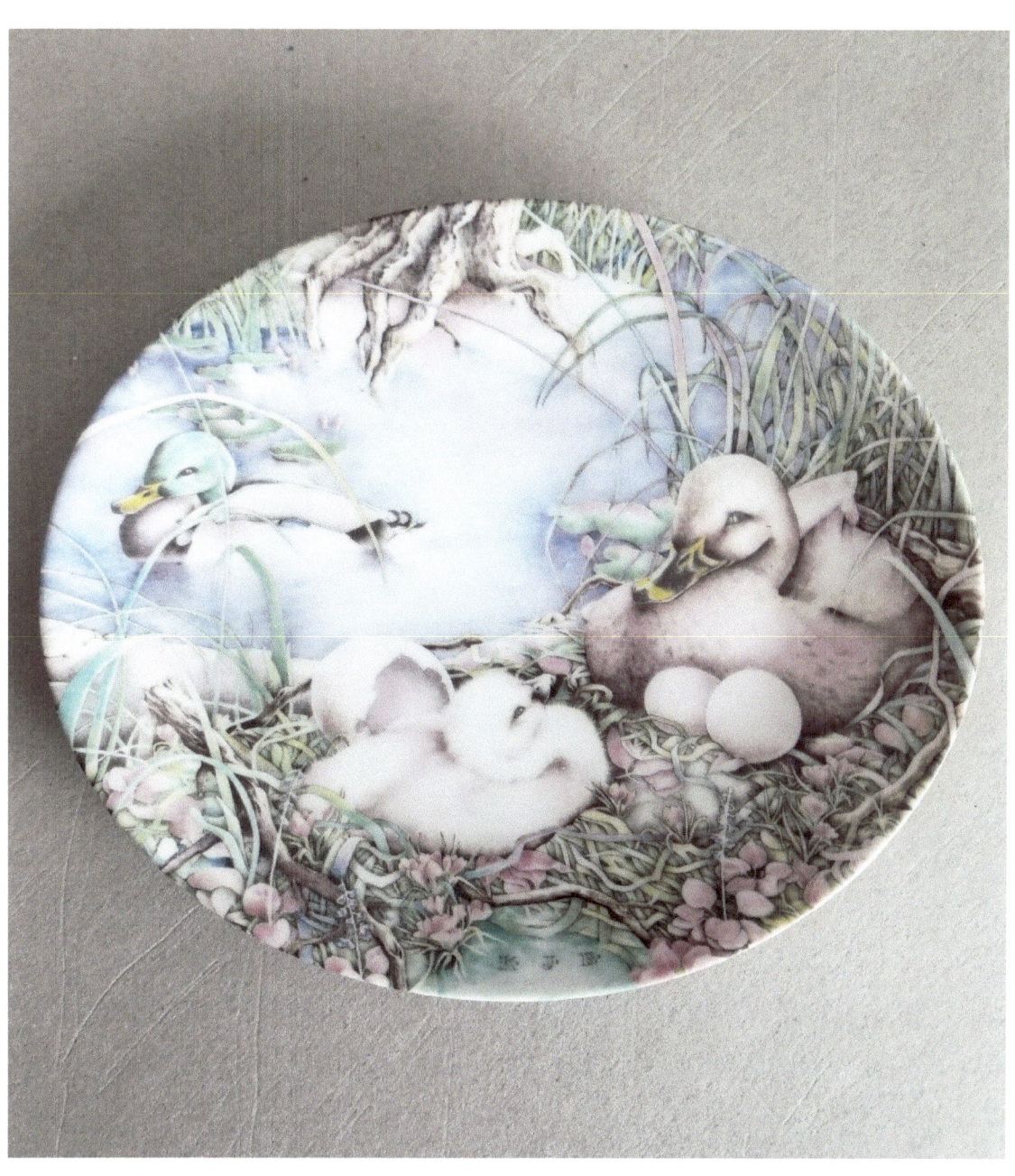

Michael J Fox

Ten percent of every book sold will go to

    The. Parkinson's Foundation

Change

People can't help a thought , but they can control their thinking.

Do you spend a lot of time thinking on things you can't do? How bad your life is?

Turn your thoughts around and think on good things.instead of thinking on what you can't do. Focus on the things you can do.

I know it is very hard to change how you think. Especially if you are suffering from (Pd).

Humor

In LA at the Mall.

There was 6 people on the elevator. Three of the them had (Pd). The other =3 were 3 ladies.shopping. There was a bump.one of the two women said.Did you feel that tremor? The 3 with (Pd) laughed...That was us

The Bible says the joy of the lord is my strength.

A merry heart does good like a medicine

Why so cast down oh my soul ? Put your hope in God

www.ingramcontent.com/pod-product-compliance
Lightning Source LLC
Chambersburg PA
CBHW051839210526
45473CB00005B/1949